Calcium Deficiency Natural Treatments: Discover Best Calcium Containing Foods

"Use calcium to build your bones and eliminate body acids"

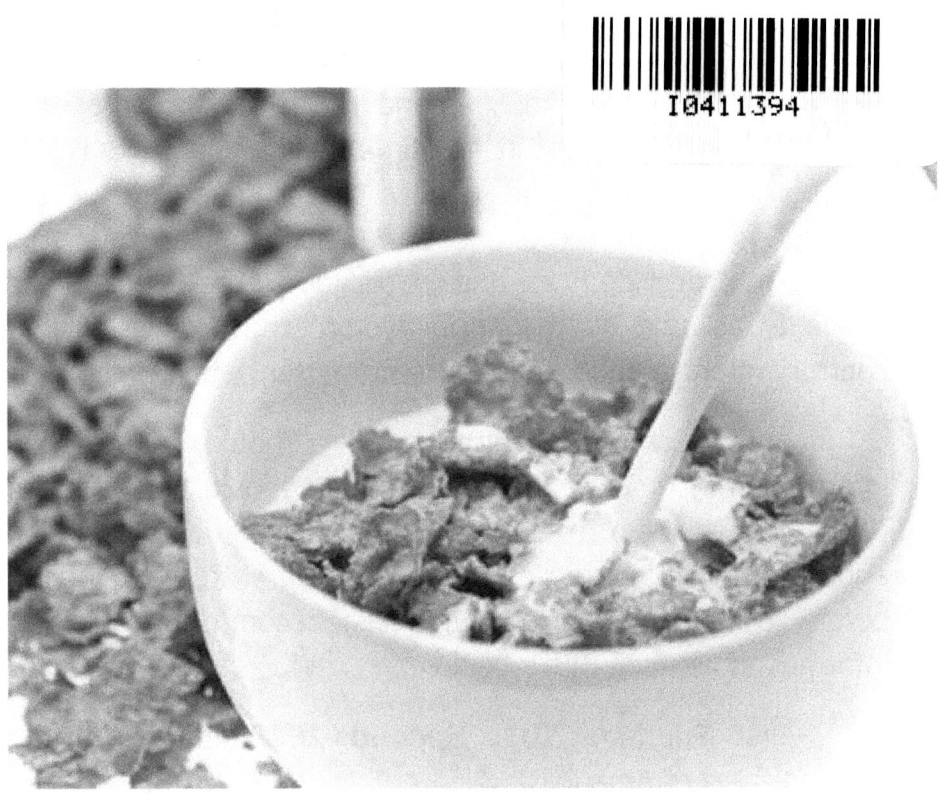

Rudy Silva, Nutritionist

Table of Contents

1: The Calcium In Your Body

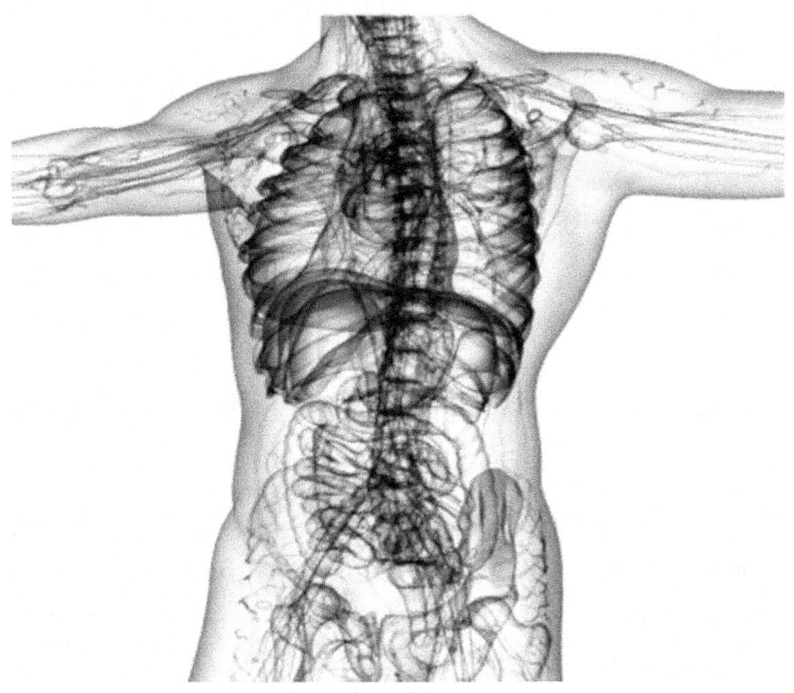

Calcium, Magnesium, D3, K2

Your body needs vitamin D3, K2, and magnesium to get calcium into your body. Without these three nutrients, you will absorb very little calcium and you will be plagued with various illnesses and you will die prematurely. Without magnesium, you can't activate the many benefits of vitamin D3. Once

This combination of these nutrients is probably one of the most important health concepts you need to get right. The power of vitamin D3 has the potential to diminish, alleviate, and prevent many of the diseases and body conditions that you suffer from.

But, keep in mind that these four nutrients are not more important than other nutrients, because a deficiency in any of the other nutrients can cause a disease. It just that calcium is the most active mineral in the body and is involved in the more biochemical reactions in your body than any other nutrient.

What is in This Book?

If you lack the body requirements of calcium, you will not be healthy. When you lack calcium, there are a number of illnesses your will contract. If you have too much calcium, this too will create poor health. This book will help you decide if you are deficient in calcium

In the following pages, you will discover how calcium, magnesium, vitamin D3, and vitamin K2 function in your body. You will find out what you need to do to make sure you are not deficient in these minerals.

Then, in the last chapter of this book, you will discover the power of vitamin D3 and vitamin K2 and how they must be used with calcium and magnesium. There are recommendations on how much of these nutrients you should be using as a group.

If you lack or have an excess of magnesium, this book will list the symptoms and diseases that you will be prone to. If you lack vitamin D, this book will help you discover how to maintain the proper levels of this vitamin. Vitamin D is the key to making sure you absorb calcium and magnesium into your blood.

The nutrients Calcium, magnesium, Vitamin K2 and

vitamin D3, work together to get the most calcium into your blood and cells.

Calcium occurs in the earth as limestone, calcium carbonate, as gypsum, or as apatite. It is always found combined with some other element. You will never find a pure calcium rock. When these types of calcium compounds combine with water, they form an alkaline solution. This is one of the reasons why you want to know as much about calcium since it is one of the main elements that can make your body liquids alkaline. One of the most important health programs you need to pursue is to move your body from an acid condition into an alkaline condition.

When your body is maintained consistently in an acid condition, calcium is also consistently removed from your bones, which results in porous bones.

Calcium is the most abundant of the minerals in your body and it makes up 1.6% of your body weight or represents 40% of all of the minerals in your body. But, 99% of the calcium you have is located in your bones. The other 1% is distributed throughout your body, and it's involved in numerous structural and biochemical processes throughout your body.

Bone Loss

Bone loss starts around middle age. For women, it increases during menopause. For men, bone loss is slow but steady starting from around 30. In bone loss, there are normally no symptoms. But, here are a few that stand out:

- Bone deformity or rickets

- Muscle and leg cramps
- Insomnia
- Growth retardation

Unfortunately, around 40% of women who live over 75 years will experience bone loss factures. Here are some reasons for low bone mass at any age.

- A diet that lacks the daily use of fruits and vegetables
- Slender body or low weight
- Premature menopause
- Anorexia nervosa
- Extreme athletic training
- Lack of exercise or a sedentary lifestyle

Excess eating or using various types of meat or protein, phosphorus, sodium, caffeine, wheat bran, and alcohol

- Smoking
- Excess use of sodas
- Use of corticosteroid medications
- Prolong bed rest or confined to a wheelchair

King of the Bioelements

It has been found that if you lack a small drop in the required level of calcium in your body this deficiency will activate aging and many degenerative diseases. Even though calcium is a large atom, it chemically moves 10,000 times faster and is 10,000 times stronger than magnesium. This gives calcium the ability to bind quickly and strongly with important biological molecules, which sustain life. This chemical flexibility gives calcium the honor of being called "the King of the Bioelements."

In this book, you will discover why it has this name. Despite there is more calcium in the body than any other mineral, with exception of oxygen, calcium is not more important than the other minerals, since all work together and are needed in your body for maintaining life.

What we can say about calcium is that it is involved in more biochemical activities in your body than any other mineral, so that it is important to supply your body with a good amount of calcium. Your body will eliminate the excess calcium from your body as its natural behavior, even when it is in a supersaturated form in your body liquids. But, when there is a deficiency of other minerals in your body that must balance with calcium, like sodium, excess calcium can react un-naturally, causing calcium crystalline deposits, which lead to pain and disease.

Calcium Crystalline Stones

Your body, when it lacks calcium and has weak or porous bones, will deposit calcium crystalline stones in various places in your body as it tries to build up weak bones. A misconception is that if you have calcium deposits in the joints or tissue giving you pain, that you have too much calcium. The truth is you do not have enough calcium, so the body tries to compensate for this by calcium deposit to build your bones back up.

Sodium-Potassium Pump

Calcium is found in your blood, bone structure, tissue,

muscles, lymph liquid, and in everybody cell in your body. It is found in the lymph liquid outside and inside your cells. In the so-called **Sodium-Potassium Pump,** the mineral sodium moves out of the cell and moves potassium into the cell. When the inside of the cell has mostly potassium, the electrical charge inside the cell is less than the charge outside of the cell where sodium dominates. This condition attracts calcium to carry food nutrients into the cell and to perform in the cells various biochemical and bioelectrical reactions.

Calcium ions also play a major role in nerve stimulation and transmission, muscle contraction and movement, and organ hormone secretion and many other biological functions. It is involved with your body's enzymes to produce energy.

Calcium ionic concentrations are the most regulated mineral in your blood plasma. Its ionic form is Ca^{++} and in this form, its most important function is in nerve function. For nerve function, calcium keeps your nerves receptive to sodium ions which help to transmit brain impulses and information to various parts of the body, which regulate your body's activities.

In those cultures where drinking water had a high content of calcium, it was found that people's lifespan was 10 years or more of the lifespan in western countries.

Kidneys

Your kidneys act as filters for your blood and they remove those nutrients or chemicals that your body no longer needs from your blood and this includes calcium. Excess calcium is routed to your bladder where it is expelled in your urine. If calcium is still needed, your kidneys will pass it into your blood to be reused by your body.

Most minerals and vitamins combine and react with calcium to produce the various body structures and chemicals that make up your body

It was thought at one time that if you produced kidney stones that you needed to take less calcium. If you tend to form kidney stones, you will have increased calcium in your urine, but this is caused by your body pulling calcium out of your bones.

Because eating excess meat cause your body to excrete calcium it is recommended, for kidney stones, to eat less meat, increase use of fruits and vegetables, supplement with calcium citrate, magnesium, vitamin B6 and vitamin C.

Take calcium citrate on an empty stomach. Most other supplements are taken with meals.

Calcium Toxicity
Usually, there is no calcium toxicity, even when you take a large dose. There is some concern that people with a tendency toward kidney stones should avoid excess calcium, but these concerns have not been proven. Kidney stores are more related to diet and those people who favor an acid diet tend to form kidney stones. In an acid diet, calcium is active and depleted as it is used up neutralizing body acids.

2: How Calcium Works In Your Body

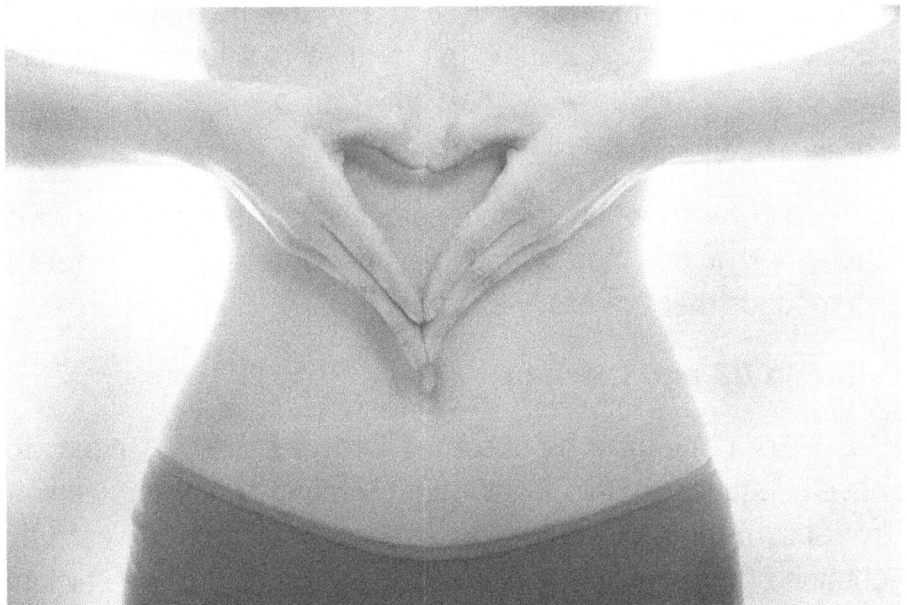

Functions of Calcium

Here is a list of some of the important biochemical and bioelectrical functions of calcium in the body:

- Absorption of calcium
- Activity in cell function
- Maintaining an alkaline body
- Contributing to Saliva alkaline body test
- Needed Calcium foods

Adsorption of Calcium

Calcium is one of the more difficult minerals to digest and to absorb through your intestinal walls.   Various phosphates and other compounds (Phosphates are derived from phosphoric acid and when they combine with oxygen they become organic phosphates, which have important biochemical activities in your body) found in red meat and sodas react with calcium to form a calcium phosphate precipitate. This prevents calcium from being absorbed and calcium is then excreted from your body.

However, when calcium comes in contact with the food substance of milk and various fruits and vegetables, it forms compounds that are easily absorbed.

Vitamin D3 and Calcium

For calcium to be absorbed into your body, it needs to have adequate vitamin D. Without Vitamin D, calcium cannot be absorbed into your bloodstream. Vitamin D can be obtained from the sun and is critical in the amount of calcium absorption that occurs in your small intestine. This is why you need to get at least 20 minutes of sun every day. In some parts of the world less time is needed and in other parts more time is needed.

You can also get vitamin D from supplements. Some foods have it but in very small quantities. When the sun's UV light hits your skin, fatty acids in your skin create vitamin D and **Inositol triphosphate, INSP-3**. This vitamin D finds its way into your intestinal wall where it assists calcium to move through your intestinal walls and into your bloodstream.

Inositol Triphosphate

Inositol triphosphate finds its way into every body cell. Its function is to release calcium from storage from within your cells when insufficient calcium is not provided by your diet and supplements, or when insufficient vitamin D causes less calcium to be absorbed in the intestinal wall.

Inositol is obtained from foods such as fruits, vegetables, grains, and from liver, kidney, and heart.

When there is insufficient calcium in the cell walls, because it got used up, the parathyroid hormone stimulated by a deficiency of vitamin D activates the extraction of calcium from your bones. Once the bones become weaken, your body starts extracting calcium from proteins that regulate your cell functions. This results in a variety of aliment and disease symptoms.

Once in your bloodstream, calcium is deposited in bones with the help of the hormone, calcitonin, released by the parathyroid gland. Also, both Calcitonin and Inositol triphosphate regulate the storage and removal of calcium within the cells. The parathyroid gland is regulated by the pituitary gland, which is right behind the eyes. When you wear sunglasses this blocks the full spectrum UV light that is needed to regulate the pituitary gland so that it can produce the hormones needed to regulate calcium in your cells.

Without adequate amounts of vitamin D, calcium will not be absorbed in proper amounts into your body and will just pass right through, excreted from your body.

Parathyroid – How it regulates calcium

The parathyroid is actively involved in maintaining your calcium blood levels. These levels are maintained to a very strict range. When your blood calcium levels drop, the parathyroid releases a hormone that directs the release of calcium from your bones and into your bloodstream. And at the same time, it tells your kidneys not to excrete calcium into your urine.

Now, when you have excess calcium in your blood, the amount of the parathyroid hormone secreted is decreased. This causes the kidney to expel more calcium into your urine. As all of this is happening, the parathyroid also releases a hormone called Calcitonin, which reduces the amount of calcium that is pull out of your bones.

Activity in cell function

Calcium is active in the process involving the Sodium-Potassium Pump in that it uses this pump to enter and exit from a cell. When it enters the cell, it brings in food nutrients to feed the cells. Once it releases these nutrients, it becomes a free ion. As these calcium ions build up in the cell, the voltage across the cell membrane will again reach 70 millivolts. This sets the stage for nutrients and toxins in the cell to be pushed out of the cell and for other nutrients to enter the cell.

Maintaining an alkaline body

The fluid outside the cells is called extracellular fluid. This fluid is maintained at a pH of 7.4 by a calcium compound called calcium mono orthophosphate. This fluid is capable of neutralizing acids that come out of the cells or arrive there from food that you have eaten. Sodium is also in the extracellular fluid and can neutralize acids, but it is needed in large quantities to maintain the Sodium-Potassium Pump cell activity. Wherever calcium is in the tissue, joints, blood, liquid or organs, it will neutralize acids.   This process reduces damage to your tissues and elevates your body pH, making it more alkaline.

When you don't have enough calcium in your body, the cells will not have enough calcium to neutralize body acids and this will cause cell deterioration and will lead to various diseases.

Keeping your body liquid alkaline or with a pH above 6.8 to 7.5 is what you should be working toward with any health program that you are working with. This can be done by using the right alkaline diet.

The Right Diet

The right diet is using both acid and alkaline foods in the right amounts. When you eat more acid foods, such as meat, butter, fats, carbohydrates, then your body needs to use up its alkaline stores to neutralize this acid, to prevent damage to your body's cells and tissue.

When you eat more alkaline foods than you need, you run the risk of not getting enough protein or carbohydrate and your pH can move above 7. 5 or 8.0 which can also lead to disease. You need a balance of certain foods to get your body pH in the range of 7.0

The saliva alkaline body test

In other my other book, "Alkaline Body," the saliva test has been discussed completely so that you can check its pH. This test is a strong indicator of whether your calcium ion level is sufficient. Here is a review. When your Saliva pH is 7.0 to 7.5 it is considered alkaline and normal. When this is the case, your urine will be slightly acidic. When you lack ionic calcium, your pH will be 4.6 to 6.4 and your urine will tend to be alkaline.

Now here is important information. If you have physical ailments, your pH will be between 6.0 to 6.5. In this case, you should take around 2000 mg of calcium rather than 1000 mg. If your pH is below 6.0, most likely, you will have various disease symptoms. And, you should be taking around 3000 mg of calcium. Once you bring up your salivary pH, you can lower your calcium intake.

If your saliva tests show your pH to be below 6.0 then by taking more calcium supplements and by eating more fruits and vegetable during the day and especially in the evening, you can change your pH to 7.0

Keep in mind that the saliva test may not always be accurate since the saliva pH can be influenced by food recently eaten. To get the most accurate reading take the saliva test only after 2 hours after your last meal or snack. Also, bring saliva into your mouth 3 times and swallow, but taking the test. Take the test 3 times on 3 different days to make sure your readings are consistent.

In my kindle e-book called "Acid Reflux: Fast and Easy Cures For Acid Reflux, Updated 2012 Version" I show you how you can change your body from 6.0 pH to 7.0 pH. In addition, in this book, I show you how to do the saliva test properly so that you can get a good reading.

Simply changing your diet, taking vitamins, and mineral supplements when you eat can change your body's pH to the 7.0 to 7.5 level. When you do this you will see a change in any physical ailment and disease that you might have. It will not occur instantly. You will need to keep this pH level for a few months.

3: Body Imbalances caused by calcium deficiency

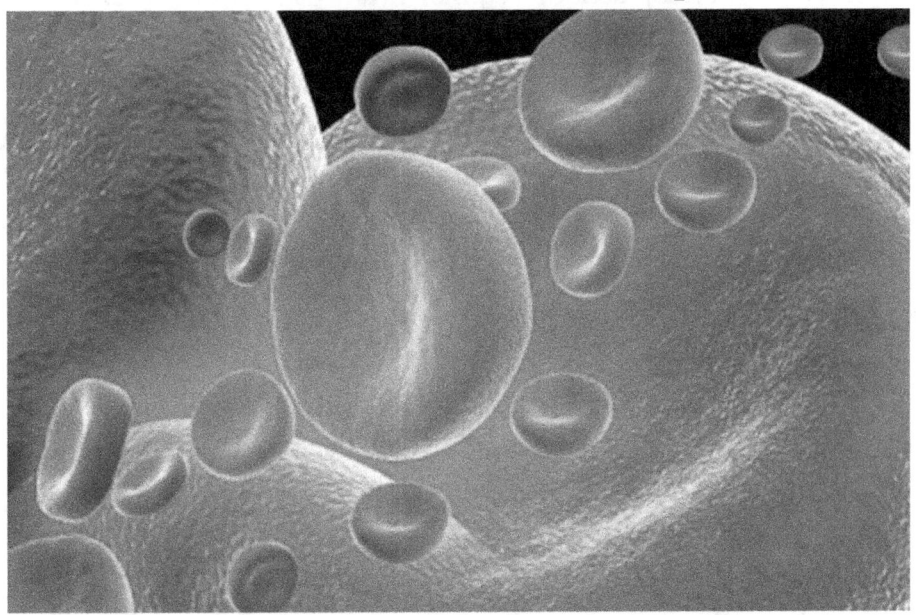

What Calcium Does in Your Body

Calcium plays a major role in blood, cells, liver, kidney, and heart health. Calcium maintains blood pH to 7.40, solidifies bones, and helps heal scars, and fights scurvy and germs. It is present in cartilage, fluids, and tissue. It is useful for Indigestion, headaches, muscle pains, arthritis, ileitis, colitis, asthma. Lack of calcium creates problems, symptoms, and disease in the areas mentioned above.

Calcium is now considered necessary to prevent cancer and should be used when you have it. The one thing to remember is that calcium from food sources does not contribute to arteriosclerosis, calcium deposits, increase blood pressure, and other illnesses.

Calcium the Healer

Calcium is one of the main minerals that promote healing in bones, tissue, organs, brain and in all parts of the body. It is carried to various parts of the body through the blood vessels. When you lack calcium, these infected or weaken areas do not get repaired properly and disease sets in. Without the necessary calcium, your body needs blood coagulation is affected and excess bleeding can occur.

Sun Glasses

Sunlight is a necessary energy that helps to ensure the absorptions of calcium. But, sunlight also plays another important role in the regulation of calcium throughout your body. Sunlight or full spectrum white light plays a major role in how the pituitary and pineal glands work. In the workplace, however, the lighting is artificial and this has a big impact on your long-term health.

The use of sunglasses is quite popular and because of the many different sunglass tints that exist, people wearing them filter out the sunlight frequencies associated with that tint. Full spectrum light, like sunlight, is necessary for proper function of the pituitary and pineal glands.

In the book, The Calcium Factor: The Scientific Secret of Health And youth, 2000, Robert R. Barefoot & Carl J. Reich, M.D. said,

"When artificial full spectrum lighting is used, human calcium absorption increases, plants flourish and cows produce 15% more milk...Tinted glasses can eliminate a large percentage of the sun's spectrum and therefore affect you both physically and psychologically. Thus, full spectrum light plays a vital role in the maintenance of the balanced hormonal system and is therefore indispensable in maintaining a balanced calcium serum."

Osteoporosis

Osteoporosis is the lack of calcium in the bone and it is estimated that over 30% of the older population will develop this condition. This is not a condition that results from old age, but a condition that comes from having an acid body for a long time.

Since the endocrine glands exert a great amount of control over calcium, the endocrine glands are put out of balance by sugar. This causes an imbalance in calcium and then shows up as cavities in your teeth.

It is the imbalance of calcium in your body that is the start of the development of chronic illnesses.

Menstrual Flow

Menstrual blood contains up to 40 times more calcium than regular blood. If you have excessive flow then you become depleted of calcium and iron. It is during this period that you should be eating kale, using liquid chlorophyll, and the many foods outlined in this e-book.

Without using a program that replaces your loss of calcium and iron during your periods, you open yourself to various diseases later on. For a diet that contains plenty of iron, you can check out my book called, "Quick and Easy Diet Cures 4 Iron Deficiency Anemia."

Teeth health

Your teeth are made up of calcium phosphate. They are kept healthy by your blood and the nutrients that you supply them. The external part of your teeth is protected by enamel, which is an extremely strong material. But, acids that form in your mouth, when sugar is eaten, create an excess of bacteria that can penetrate the enamel.

Having dental cavities is a sign of a lack of calcium. When your body needs calcium and you have not provided enough in your diet or your calcium body stores are depleted, calcium is pulled out of your teeth and bones to bring your body back into calcium balance. This weakens the teeth and bacteria can penetrate the enamel causing tooth decay.

Arteriosclerosis

Arteriosclerosis is not caused by an excess of calcium. It is caused by the lack of sodium and chlorine salts. Calcium needs these salts to be properly used and to stay in solution and not precipitate out onto artery walls. It is needed so that artery walls don't become inflamed by acid damage and consequently need repair through plaque buildup.

Arteriosclerosis occurs when plaque builds up along the artery walls, which takes place over years. Eventually, this plaque will narrow the arteries and cause reduced blood flow or blood flow blockage. Reduced blood flow will result in many different illnesses because cells will not be getting the proper oxygen and nutrition. This blockage will result in heart attacks.

Plaque is made up of phospholipids, collagen,

triglycerides, fibrin mucopolysaccharides, cholesterol, heavy metals, proteins, muscle tissue, and debris, which is all bonded by calcium.

Plaque only occurs in arteries that deliver blood from the heart to your body and not in the veins that return blood to the heart. Cholesterol is not the cause of plaque, but even if it was it can be controlled by diet and not drugs. Eighty percent of the cholesterol in your body is created in the body and 20% of it comes from your diet. Your body uses cholesterol in every cell, in hormones, in nerve impulses, in the brain, and in the creation of vitamin D on your skin.

It is the cellular breakdown along the artery walls caused by acidity surrounding the wall tissue that prompts repair of that area and that is when plaque starts to build up on the wall.

Heart Disease

Calcium is a central to good heart function. Since the calcium ion is linked to proper cell function any deterioration in the cell do the lack of calcium will affect the cell structure of heart cells and to the cells of the arteries. This deterioration will lead to heart diseases.

In addition, the ability of the heart to contract and expand is due to the ionization of calcium – Ca++.

Effects Of Excess Calcium

When your body has an excess of calcium, you will see external and internal boney growths. These growths can occur in any part of your bodies such as joints, tissue, organs, or muscle. The growths may appear as kidney stones or other precipitates that occur on your heels, shoulder joints, knee joints, or toe bones.

Calcium and magnesium need to be in a certain balance to prevent lack of blood calcium. Studies have shown that it is best to have a calcium to magnesium ratio of 1:1. Past recommendations have been a 2:1 ratio.

When you have excess calcium, you need to eat more fruits and vegetables to get the natural absorbable vitamins and minerals, especially sodium. Sodium and calcium must always be in balance, lack of one or the other leads to a chemical imbalance, which results in various illnesses or diseases.

Illness or Conditions Due To Lack Of Calcium

Here some of the symptoms or conditions that occur when you lack calcium:

- tumors
- sores, abscesses, inflammations
- discharges
- deformed fingers, bones, hips cranial bones
- tooth decay
- undersized organs
- blood deficiencies
- back pain
- vomiting
- tuberculosis
- excess bleeding

- excess mucus discharge
- poor scar healing
- craving for salt
- bone softening
- swelling knuckles
- bronchial congestion
- wrinkled skin
- cystic goiter
- cyst formation
- nervous problems

There are so many illness and poor body conditions that occur when you lack calcium. You may on have a few of these, but if they are consistent and they remain with you for a while, consider increasing your calcium intake.

Nervous Problems

Anxiety is supposed to help you when you are involved in stressful or life threating situation. Under these conditions your metabolism increases, muscles tighten, and you get a shot of adrenaline. When anxiety happens, you do use up many minerals and that includes calcium. Under stressful conditions that last more than a day, it is wise to take a calcium supplement.

Back pain

Back pain is one of those conditions that when it occurs it can disable you and cause you to take a quick trip to the emergency. When back pain is caused by strained muscles, stress, bad posture, inactivity, or lack of exercise, one of the supplements recommend is calcium with magnesium. These minerals reduce muscle spasms, muscle tightness, and nerve irritation.

Taking a supplement that contains calcium, magnesium, and vitamin D daily will help to alleviate this long list of body conditions or illnesses. Just remember that calcium is a relaxer and nerve reliever.

4: Eating calcium foods

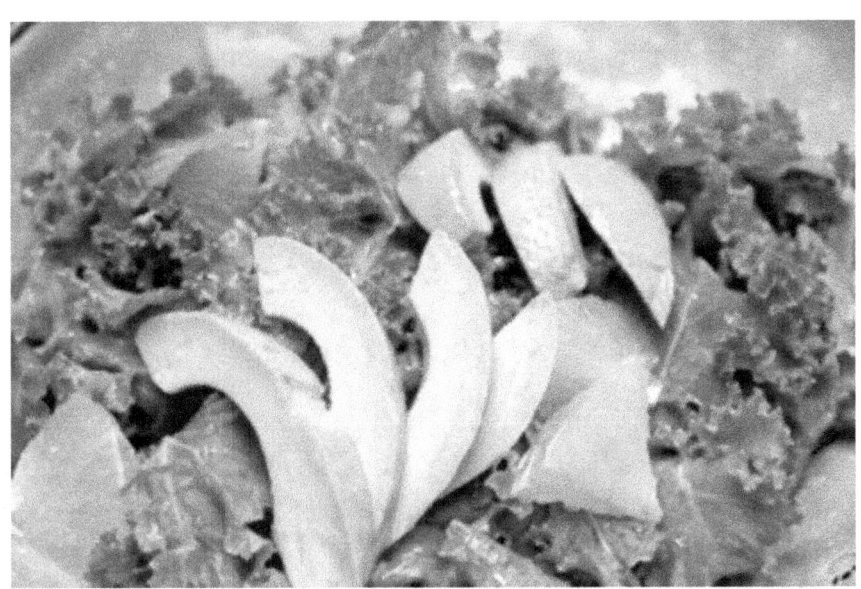

Calcium absorption

Even though you eat calcium foods, only around 25% of the calcium in this food will be absorbed by your body. But, as a child or if you are pregnant, you may absorb up to 60%.

When cooking fruits or vegetables, you should use lower temperatures, when possible. When produce is heated to above 150 Fahrenheit at least 33% of the available calcium is lost.

Calcium and Milk

All milk that is pasteurized at high temperature is a low source of calcium. There is some milk that is pasteurized at 145 degrees Fahrenheit that are better sources of calcium. All milk that has been pasteurized or homogenized is acidic. The best milk source for calcium is raw goat milk and since it has not been heated it is alkaline in nature.

Despite the insistence from The Dairy Council that,

"Milk has been part of the diet for thousands of years. Despite the fact that milk is one of the most nutritionally complete foods available, there are many myths relating to consumption that blame milk and dairy foods for a variety of ailments. Many of these myths have been part of the folklore for centuries and are not founded on science."

There is a tremendous amount of scientific papers and finding that milk should not be included in your diet because of the illnesses it contributes too. But, then again there are studies that show there is a decrease in heart and cancer in people that drink milk. Just remember milk is an acid food and has to be balanced off with alkaline food.

An article, In 1992 The New England Journal of Medicine pointed out that, "Consumption of cow's milk has been associated with insulin-dependent diabetes..."

But, this is also evidence that some milk should be drunk and that there are other sources of dairy products that can provide plenty of calcium for your diet, such as yogurt or cottage cheese.

Because of the tremendous activity of calcium in the body in relation to cell nutrition and its alkalizing effect, it is best to eat plenty of those vegetables and fruits that are high in calcium.

In his book, **Prescription for Natural Cures**, 2004, by James F. Balch, M.D. he says,

"It may surprise you to learn that countries, where people drink the most milk, are also those with the highest rates of osteoporosis. This may be due to the fact that lactose intolerance and casein allergy are very common and lead to malabsorption. Also, calcium from cow's milk is not well absorbed, at a rate of 25 percent. Milk products lead to other health problems as well, so don't rely on them as source calcium. Unsweetened, cultured yogurt is an exception."

One way to eat your unsweetened yogurt is to add it to a blender and then add fruits like strawberries, pineapple, mango, bananas, and so on. To get add additional sweetness, you can add some raw honey, since honey helps you to absorb

The British Medical Research Council made a 10-year study of 5000 men aged 45 to 59. In this study they found,

"Only 1 percent of those who regularly drank more than one-half liter of milk a day suffered heart attacks ... against 10 percent of those who drank no milk at all."

In this study, researchers also found there was no difference whether they drank pure milk or skimmed, the benefits were still there.

There is still a lot of controversy about drinking milk for calcium. If you feel good drinking milk, then you should drink it. If you develop mucus or other symptoms when you drink milk, then you should consider getting your calcium from other sources.

Where you can get calcium

One of the highest sources of calcium comes from **barley, green kale,** and **turnip greens**. You can get good calcium from cereals and grains.

Here is a list of foods highest in calcium:

- Seaweed – dulse, kelp, Irish moss, wakame, nori, kombu, agar
- Sardines with bones
- Tempeh, tofu
- Avocados, figs, prunes
- All dark greens, collard greens, spinach, kale,
- Unprocessed seeds and nuts – sesame seeds, grains, and nuts, almonds, walnuts
- Bone Broth
- Cows, skimmed milk, cheese, cottage cheese, goat milk, yogurt
- Rice milk-calcium enriched
- Cabbage, cauliflower, celery, lemons, rhubarb
- Egg yolk, gelatin foods
- Fish, meat near the bone
- Whole wheat bread
- Beans, brown rice, lentils, millet, oats,
- Broccoli, Brussels sprouts, cauliflower
- Onions, parsnips, watercress

- Raw butter, gelatin, blackstrap molasses
- Coconut, raw cream, egg yolk
- Fish, meat near the bone, bone broth
- Natural cane sugar

The amount of calcium in certain foods

½ cup of wakame – sea vegetable gives 1700 mg

¼ cup of agar – sea vegetable gives 1000 mg

½ cup of nori – sea vegetable gives 600 mg

¼ cup of kombu – sea vegetable gives 500 mg

1 cup of tempeh gives 340 mg

8 oz. of calcium enriched rice milk give 300 mg

1 cup of almonds gives 300 mg

8 oz. of skim milk gives 302 mg

8 oz. of low-fat yogurt gives 300 mg

1 oz. of Swiss cheese gives 272 mg

10 figs give 269 mg

½ cup of tofu gives 258 mg

½ cup of sesame seeds gives 250 mg

1 oz. of mozzarella cheese gives 183 mg

½ cup of boiled collards gives 179 mg

1 tablespoon of blackstrap molasses gives 172 mg

1 cup cottage cheese gives 126 mg

2 sardines in oil give 92 mg

¼ cup of walnuts gives 70 mg

1 cup of black beans or lentils give 55 mg

½ cup of boiled mustard greens gives 52 mg

½ cup of boiled broccoli gives 36 mg

Dark Greens

The dark greens can be boiled instead of steamed and their taste is improved. Boiling them also does not cause them to reduce their nutritional value since they have such high nutrition, to begin with.

Meat

Limit the amount of meat you eat. Meat has 30 times more phosphorous than calcium. And, in the digestive tract, this phosphorous will cause the calcium to precipitate to form apatite, which is a form of phosphorous calcium mineral crystal. It is apatite that is the substance that forms your bones. This result is that this calcium is not available to you and is excreted from your body.

Sugar

It has been found that there is 40% less calcium in white sugar as compared to raw sugar. Blackstrap molasses has 258 times more calcium as white sugar. Calcium and sugar attract each other. The more sugar you eat the more calcium is precipitated. The less body calcium you have the more tooth decay you will have.

Salt

Using excess salt in your food has been associated with bone loss. If you eat salt with your food, salt competes with calcium to get absorbed. The more salt is absorbed the less calcium is. Try using culinary herbs and chili sauces to flavor your food.

If you like salty food, you could use them as a snack and not with your regular meals.

Nightshades

Foods like tomatoes, potatoes, eggplant, peppers, and tobacco, which are considered nightshade foods.

In her book, Food and Healing, 1986, Annemarie Colbin points out that,

"In my own experience and that of some of my students, consuming nightshades on a dairy-free diet has resulted in a loss of calcium, evidenced by brittle nails, painful gums, and dental caries. Eliminating the nightshades, rather than increasing the dairy, solved the problem"

There are some foods that promote the excretion of calcium. We have indicated that eating excess meat can trap calcium and eliminate it from your body. Foods high in oxalic acid also promote the removal of calcium from your body – spinach, cranberries, and rhubarb.

Wheat bran also limits the amount of calcium you absorb because of the phytic acid in its fiber. The phytic acid in wheat fiber has the ability to combine with calcium and limit its absorption in your body.

Other things that limit your calcium absorption are eating too many foods that contain phosphorus, drinking tea which contains tannins, lack of vitamin D, and having diarrhea.

Pumpkin Seeds

Shelled pumpkin seeds are a high source of zinc, magnesium, iron phosphorus, and calcium. You can eat a hand full every day.

5: Calcium Supplements that Prevent Disease

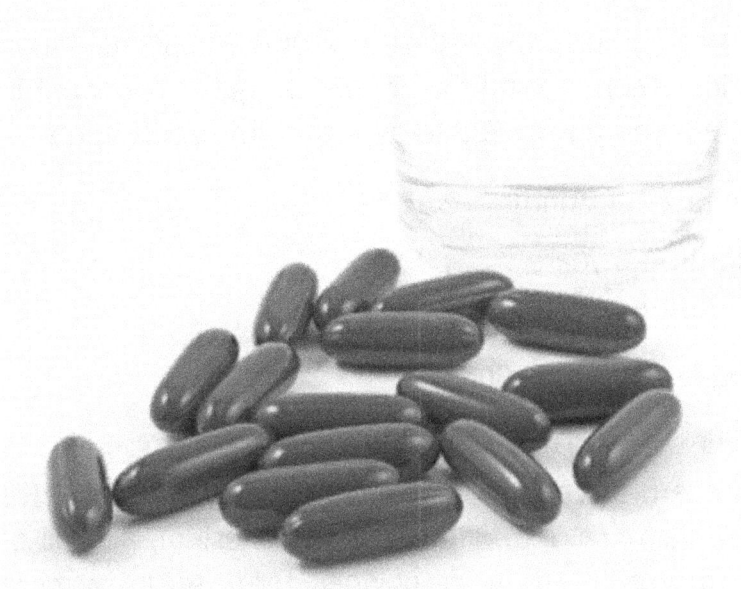

Calcium Supplements

Taking calcium supplements is a great idea since you are probably not getting all of the calcium you need in your diet. However, since calcium tends to interfere with the absorption of other minerals, it is best to also take a multivitamin that provides those other minerals.

What type of calcium supplements should you take? A good supplement is one that contains:

- Calcium 1000 – 1500 mg
- Magnesium 400 – 600 mg
- Vitamin D in Cholecalciferol form, called D3

So what are your daily requirements for calcium? Daily requirements for calcium are between 1000 to 1500mg. The type of supplement and the amount you take depends on your ability to absorb calcium. This is difficult to determine, so it is best to take the high end of calcium – 1500 mg

Here are some minimum calcium supplementation requirements. Keep in mind that if you can get this amount in your food then you don't need to take calcium supplements.

- Infants 7-12 months   270 mg
- Children 4-8 years   800mg
- Males 31-50   1000mg
- Females 31-50   1000mg
- Pregnant and lactating 1000mg

One of the best calcium supplements to use is Brazil Live Coral. It contains calcium, vitamin D, magnesium, and all of the trace minerals. It is in powder form so it is more absorbable. It contains the vitamin D you need to absorb the calcium. But, you also need to spend at least 20 to 30 minutes in the sun to get the natural vitamin D. It does not have to be in the direct sunlight, but it is better if you can do it. Look on the internet for:

Brazil Live Coral
Also look for **Okinawa coral calcium** which is another good product.

Another excellent calcium supplement is called, **3-Way Calcium Complex™**. Look for this on the internet. It uses three different forms of calcium and includes other nutrients that help you absorb more of this calcium.

Calcium absorption

For calcium to be absorbed into the body, it is crucial to have adequate vitamin D in your body. Without Vitamin D, calcium cannot be absorbed into your body. Vitamin D can be obtained from the sun and from supplements. Be aware that wearing sunglasses can affect your health by not keeping your pituitary gland healthy.

It's the pituitary gland that tells the parathyroid to release hormones that help to regulate and absorb calcium. In addition to eating calcium foods, take Brazil Live Coral Calcium and also add vitamin D as a supplement to your diet, especially if you don't go out into the sun every day.

Vitamin C

It is believed that by taking vitamin C with Calcium, you increase the absorption of calcium. A form of calcium that is already combined with vitamin C is called Calcium Ascorbate. This type of calcium is easily transported across the intestinal walls.

Chelated calcium

It is best to use calcium supplements in chelated form. What this means is that calcium is tied to an amino acid and this makes it easier for calcium to pass through your intestinal walls. Chelated calcium is more easily absorbed than calcium that is not chelated. Here are some of the types of calcium amino acid chelates you should look for and buy.

- Calcium Alpha Keto Glutarate

- Calcium ascorbate – a form of calcium that is tied to vitamin C
- Calcium Lactate
- Calcium Alginate
- Calcium hydroxyapatite – the type of calcium found in your bones
- Calcium Glycinate
- Calcium Amino Acid Chelate
- Calcium Caprylate
- Calcium Malate
- Calcium Gluconate
- Calcium L-Aspartate
- Calcium Lactate Gluconate
- Calcium Lysinate
- Calcium Orotate
- Calcium Succinate
- Tricalcium phosphate – the type of calcium in your bones

All of these amino acids tied to calcium can also be attached to the other minerals like magnesium and potassium. So you can find magnesium alginate or magnesium alginate or magnesium aspartate.

Honey

It has been found by the United States Department of Agriculture nutritionist Richard J. Wood that the glucose in honey can increase your absorption of calcium by up to 25%. It can also increase the absorption of zinc and magnesium.

Types of Calcium to avoidCalcium Dolomite

Avoid using dolomite as a source of calcium, since it may not be absorbed properly by your body. Dolomite is a form of calcium carbonate and magnesium.

Calcium carbonate

Calcium carbonate is hard to absorb when the pH in your stomach is not at the proper level. If you low levels of stomach acid you will not be able to absorb this type of calcium.

Magnesium

Magnesium is usually found in calcium supplements because is required for proper calcium metabolism. Magnesium has a role in the formation of bones. It has been found that when there is a decrease in blood magnesium that there is also a drop in blood calcium. The lack of magnesium in your body can increase the risk of osteoporosis.

Magnesium's absorption is enhanced by vitamin D just like calcium is. Magnesium is active in making sure that cells function properly by moving sodium and potassium in and out of the cells. Magnesium, just like calcium, is important for nerve and heart function. Many of the foods that are high in calcium are also high in magnesium.

6: Alkaline Body, Saliva Test

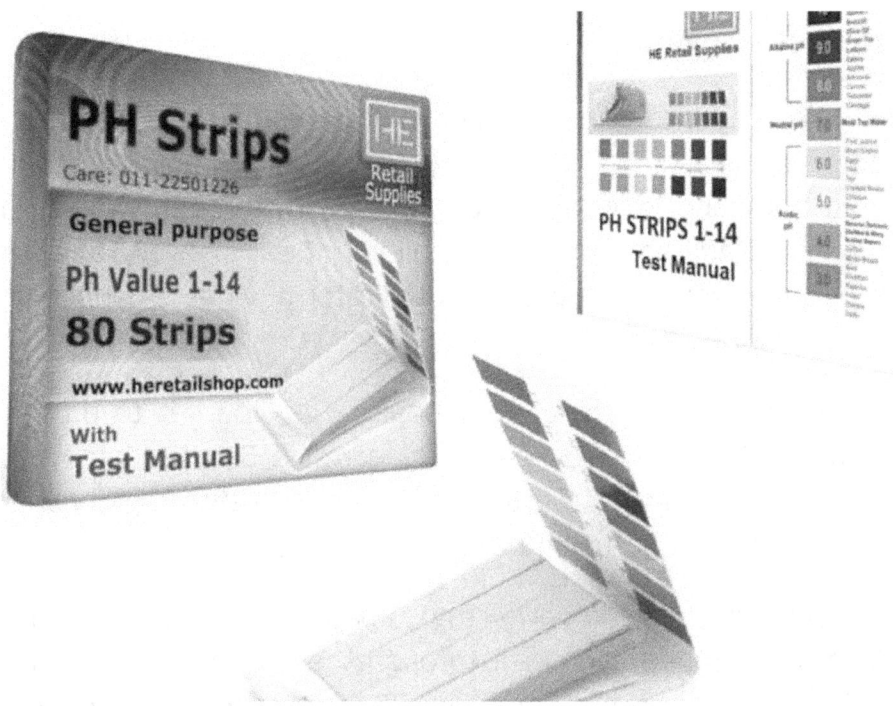

An alkaline diet helps you balance the level of acid and alkaline in all parts of your body. When you eat more acid foods, such as meat, butter, fats, carbohydrates, then your body will use up its alkaline stores to neutralize then acid residue created by these foods.

When you eat more alkaline foods than you need, you run the risk of not getting enough protein or carbohydrate and your pH can move above 7. 5 to 8.0. A high alkaline pH, 6.0 to 8.0 can also lead to disease. You need a balance of certain foods to get your body's pH in the range of 7.0

The saliva alkaline body test

In the kindle book called "Alkaline Body," the saliva test has been discussed in greater detail. This test is a strong indicator of whether your calcium ion level is sufficient.

Here is a review

You can measure the saliva in your mouth and get a fairly accurate measure of the pH in your body. Saliva is created in your body and is brought into your mouth through two saliva glands. Your body produces gallons of saliva every day, so measuring your saliva is a good indicator of what is happening inside your body.

Wait at least a couple of hours after you eat to do this saliva test. When you start, bring saliva 3 times into your mouth and swallow. On the 4th time, wet a strip of pH paper in your mouth and pull it out. Now, you can read it.

(Purchase some pH litmus paper at a drug store, laboratory outlet or order it through the Internet. The better pH paper you can buy comes in .25 increments in pH change. You can buy this litmus paper on Amazon.)

When your Saliva pH is between 6.8 to 7.4 it is considered alkaline and normal. When this is the case, your **urine** will be slightly acidic and in the range of 5.5 to 6.5. When you lack ionic calcium, your saliva pH will be 4.6 to 6.4 and your urine will even more acidic.

Now here is important information on your saliva test.

- If you have physical ailments, your pH will be from 6.0 to 6.7. In this case, you should take around 2000 mg of calcium rather than 1000 mg.

- If your pH is below 5.0 to 6.0, most likely, you will have various disease symptoms. And, you should be taking around 3000 mg of calcium. Once you bring up your salivary pH, you can lower your calcium intake.

If your saliva tests show your pH to be below 6.0, then by taking more calcium supplements and by eating more fruits and vegetable during the day and especially in the evening, you can change your pH to 6.8 to 7.4

Keep in mind that the saliva test may not always be accurate since the saliva pH can be influenced by food recently eaten. To get the most accurate reading, take the saliva test 2 hours after eating your last meal or snack. Take the test 3 times on 3 different days to make sure your readings are consistent. In my kindle e-book called "Alkaline Body," it shows you how you can change your body from 6.0 to 7.4 pH.

Simply by changing your diet, taking vitamins, and mineral supplements when you eat, you can change your body's pH to the 7.0 to 7.4 level. When you do this, you will see a change in any physical ailment and disease that you might have. It will not occur instantly. You will need to keep this pH level for a few months.

In the past, it was said that you did not need to take supplements. You could get all the nutrition your body needed from the food you ate. Today is a different story. The food supply lacks nutrients and most food in the grocery store is processed and junk food. And, it is necessary to supplement your diet with supplements or expect to develop some form of illness.

Another Saliva Test

Here is another way to approach your saliva test. This was outlined in my Alkaline Body ebook.

Saliva Test

Here is a simple test you can perform on your saliva that will give you an idea of where you stand with your body's pH level. Your saliva contains mineral salts that keep it alkaline at 6.8 to 7.4. If your body is deficient in alkaline food or minerals, it will take the minerals from your saliva causing it to drop in pH.

If your saliva is below normal, you can influence your saliva's pH to read higher, by eating more acid binding (acid binding food will be explained in the next chapter) food and by supplementing with potassium, magnesium, and calcium.

Keep in mind there are some inaccuracies with this method since your body fluids are always in transition. This test simply gives you an idea of what your saliva pH is at that moment. Use this information for your own education. Then as you begin to change your eating habits and lifestyle, you can retest to see if there is a difference.

Many doctors deny the accuracy or use of this saliva test and say it is of no value. Frankly, they prefer you to pay them a visit, so that they can put you under their care.

In an article written by Dr. Steven Zodkoy, A Free and Simple Test for pH, a Potential Health Tester, Dr. Zodkoy recommends using the saliva pH test to determine the state of your body's pH.

By testing your pH regularly, you can decide the validity of using pH litmus paper to determine the level of your health. As you make changes, you can test your saliva and urine to see if the pH litmus color changes.

You need to take this test for 3 days and at least 3 times a day and to get an average value so you can establish a baseline or a starting point for yourself.

Purchase some pH litmus paper at a drug store, laboratory outlet or order it through the Internet. The better pH paper you can buy strips with a .25 increment in pH change.

Starting Your Saliva Testing
Gather saliva in your mouth then swallow. Do this three times.

Place the pH paper under your tongue. Let it sit there for 5 seconds to wet it and then remove it. Let it sit for 10 to 20 seconds, compare the color of your pH paper to the color chart on the bottle and record the pH.

Do this test around one hour before eating or around two hours after eating. This reading gives you an idea about the state of your saliva. Your first test should be done first thing in the morning before you rinse out your mouth or drink anything.

Saliva and Lemon Test

Now, do this test immediately after you do your saliva test above. Squeeze the juice of half a lemon into one ounce of water, and swish it around in your mouth for 5 seconds or so. Then spit it out, wait one minute, now, measure your mouth's pH with litmus paper. Just place the paper into your mouth and wet it.

Now compare the color and pH value of this reading with your first pH saliva reading. This reading should have a higher alkaline reading than your first saliva reading.

Good Saliva Test

If this reading has a higher alkaline reading, it means you have alkaline reserves. The higher the alkaline reading you have the stronger your alkaline reserves. A small alkaline upward change means you have alkaline reserves, but they are not as strong as they should be.

For example,

- Morning reading is 6.5 pH
- After the lemon test reading 6.9 pH

These readings are good and indicate you have some alkaline mineral stores. But, your Morning reading of 6.5 is a little low and should be closer to 6.8 to 7.0 for better health.

Weak Saliva Test

If your pH reading does not change from your first reading or actually goes down, by becoming more acidic, then your alkaline reserves are weak. You need to make some major changes in the way you eat. In this course, you will see what you need to do to bring up your alkaline reserves so that you will not be susceptible to serious diseases.

Now, suppose your readings were,

- First reading 6.5

- Lemon test reading 6.2

There is a drop in your lemon pH test, and this is not good. This means that you don't have enough minerals in your body to neutralize the acid in your mouth. You will have to eat more acid binding food.

Saliva Test Summary

Again, if your lemon test readings have a higher pH reading than your first reading, it means you have alkaline reserves. The bigger the difference between your first test and second test, the stronger your alkaline reserves. A small alkaline upward change means you have alkaline reserves, but they are not as strong as they should be.

If your lemon pH reading does not change from your first reading or actually goes down by becoming more acidic, then your alkaline reserves are weak, and you need to make some major changes in the way you eat. This also means you have a highly acidic body that can create some serious illness, especially if your lemon test pH is down to 6.0 and below.

7: Increase Calcium Absorption with D3

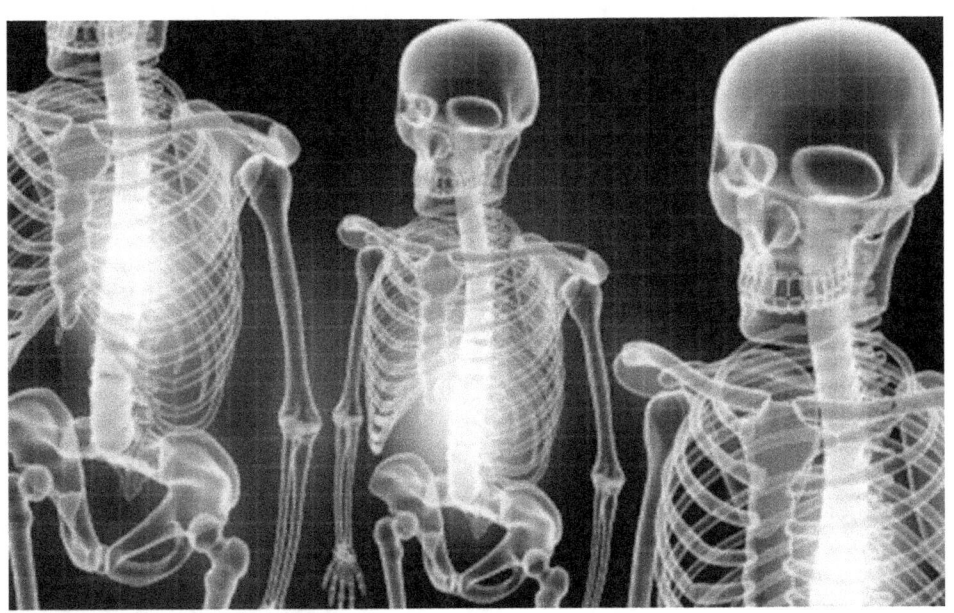

Vitamin D3, the Hormone

Vitamin D3 is considered a hormone and not a vitamin. It was mislabeled a vitamin, during the time it was discovered, since it was thought to come from food. The vitamin form that is active in your body is Vitamin D3, known as cholecalciferol. Vitamin D3 is tasked with communicating with your DNA. It turns on and off over 1000 genes to activate their function.

There is also vitamin D2, which is considerably less active in your body. D3 is around 300% more active in your body than D2. Most foods that are fortified with vitamin D use the D2 form.

Vitamin D3 is created when UV light activates a conversion form of cholesterol, which occurs in or on your skin.

D3 Helps Absorb Calcium

Another vitamin D3 function is to help you absorb calcium. Calcium aside from helping to form bone structures is a key mineral in helping to keep your body alkaline. An alkaline body is the natural state of your body, and an acid body is a state of disease. You can gain more information on how to maintain an alkaline body in my ebook called "**Alkaline Body**"

How Much Vitamin D3 do You Need?

So, what is the dose for vitamin D3? During the 30's and 40's studies showed that taking more than 50,000 IU was still safe. However, pharmaceuticals went on a scare tactic by saying that taking more than 400 IU of vitamin D was toxic.

Yet, being out in the sun for 30 minutes can produce 10,000 to 20,000 IU of vitamin D3.

When vitamin D3 was demonized during the 40's, the pharmaceuticals came out with three miracle drugs for treating various deadly diseases. These drugs were nothing more than 50,000 IU of vitamin D.

The amount of vitamin D3 you may need will depend on a couple of factors. The more obese you are the more D3 you need. You can experiment on how much you need by seeing what result you get with different doses. Take a certain amount in 3 to 4 weeks to see if your health improves.

You can start as follows:

- Normal weight – 5,000 to 10,000 IU
- Overweight – 8,000 to 12,000
- Obese – 8,000 to 15,000

If you take over 10,000 IU of vitamin D3, you will have to supplement with vitamin 1000 mcg of K2 to avoid calcium depositing in body tissue and joints.

You should be ok to take up and more than 20,000 IU of vitamin D3. To do this you must take a minimum of 1000 mcg of vitamin K2 per 10,000 IU of vitamin D3. Be sure not to take too much K2, since it can cause a racing heart or high blood pressure. If this happens, you would then just back off on the K2, until those symptoms disappear.

Doses of 8,000 IU, in studies, did not exhibit excess calcium in the blood. The additional calcium brought into the blood by high D3 supplementation was found to be properly used by the body.

Because D3 is fat soluble, you can optimize its adsorption by taking a healthy fat with it.

Calcium, Vitamin D3, and K2

Vitamin D3 helps to move calcium passed your small intestinal barrier and into your blood. Vitamin K2 then moves the calcium to the right areas of your body. K2 prevents calcium from building up along your arteries and accumulating in your soft tissue and bones. Recent studies show that K2 is beneficial in the treatment of rheumatoid arthritis. K2 is also known improving blood clotting.

Types of Vitamin K

There are several kinds of vitamin K. There are K1 and K2, where K2 has several forms of which K7 is the most active and important form. K2 (MK-4) has also shown to be beneficial for rheumatoid arthritis, RA. However, since K7 is more bioavailable then MK-4, it is the better choice for treating RA.

Aside from vitamin D3 being necessary for proper calcium absorption, strong bones, teeth, immune system, heart health, it is also useful in the prevention of cancer and other diseases. Low levels of Vitamin D3 are associated with almost every disease you develop.

In the NaturalHealth365 website article, Lori Alton, staff writer, writes,

"According to the Institute of Medicine, 4,000 IU daily is the tolerable upper level of intake – defined as the highest level that would be unlikely to cause harm to nearly all adults. However, the Vitamin D Council recommends that adults take 5,000 IU of the vitamin a day.

Meanwhile, a naturopathic practitioner might advise dosages in the area of 8,000 IU of vitamin D a day, depending on the individual's history and lifestyle. The Endocrine Society Practice Guidelines maintain that adults can safely take up to 10,000 IU a day – more than double what the IOM advises as the safe upper level.

Bottom line: ensuring that you have adequate levels of vitamin D3 just might be one of the most important things you can do to protect your health – and your life."

The supplement to take is one that has calcium, magnesium, vitamin D3, and vitamin K. If you can't find such a supplement, build one from single nutrients. To enhance the effectiveness of vitamin D3, take fish or coconut oil pill.

Alzheimer's' Disease

Low levels of body vitamin D3 have been associated with a higher risk of Alzheimer's' Disease. In addition, other diseases such as cancer (colon, prostate), respiratory infections, multiple sclerosis, and Parkinson's disease have also been associated with low D3 blood levels.

Simply by increasing your blood levels of D3, you give yourself protection against these diseases. Optimum blood levels of D3 are **50 ng/ml to 80 ng/ml**

Respiratory Infections

In a study made at Queen Mary University in London, researchers found that Vitamin D3 was just as effective as getting a flu shot in protecting against a respiratory infection. It was found that Vitamin D3 produces over 210 antimicrobials.

Immune System

It has been discovered that Vitamin D receptors have been found in all immune cells. Further studies show that various autoimmune disorders benefit from increased Vitamin D3 supplementation.

Heart Disease

Low levels of blood vitamin D3 have been associated with

cardiovascular and stroke issues. Higher levels of D3 are related to the lowest risks of heart attack, stroke, and death.

Magnesium

Magnesium is necessary for calcium to function properly in your body. It also activates enzymes that help your body use vitamin D3. Without magnesium, vitamin D3 cannot be used by your body. For this reason, it is not a good idea to take calcium without magnesium, vitamin D3, and vitamin K2.

To get many of the other minerals that aid in the proper function of calcium, D3, and K2, eat those foods that are high in magnesium.

You should also supplement with magnesium. The supplements to use are

Nutrients Needed by Vitamin D3

There are many other nutrients that interact with D3. These can come from your diet. Vitamin A, zinc, and boron are few important ones.

Food That Has D3

Very little D3 is found in food. The foods that have some D3 are eggs, wild cold water fish, and organic mushrooms, soy (non-GMO), unsweetened yogurt, and ricotta cheese.

Final Words on Vitamin D3

Many studies have been done on vitamin D3 and have substantiated the need to use it in doses up to 10,000 IU or more. The recommended RDA of 400 IU is totally out of line with the body's need for this vitamin, especially if you are sick.

In combination with calcium, magnesium, and K2, vitamin D3 immerges as the nutrient required in large quantities necessary for quality health.

Studies have shown that healthy blood levels of Vitamin D3 are in the range of 50 to 80 ng/ml. Blood level below 30 ng/ml has always shown to be associated with all kinds of disease. The amount of vitamin D3 required for good health has been established to be 5,000 to 10,000 IU of vitamin D3.

Here are the recommended supplement program by Robert R. Barefoot, Nutritionist and Biochemist, as stated in his 2002 book, Death by Diet.

The pH listed below is based on your saliva test listed in this book.

pH	calcium	magnesium	vit. D3	vit. A
6.5 to 7.4	1200mg	690mg	2400IU	30000IU
6.0 to 6.5	2400mg	1380mg	4800IU	60000IU
4.5 to 6.0	3600mg	2070mg	7200IU	90000IU

The pH listed in the above chart is associated with the following body conditions.

- pH 6.5 to 7.4 is the normal body condition
- pH 6.0 to 6.5 is where the body is developing a disease
- pH 4.5 to 6.0 is where you have a disease

Vitamin K

If you take less than 10,000 mg of vitamin D3, you may not need to take any vitamin K. But, if you are taking 10,000 IU or more you should take 1000mcg of K2 with some 100mcg of k7. The k7 is much stronger than the K1 or K2.

Side effects of Vitamin K

Some people have to experience Vitamin K side effects when they have taken too much. These side effects are high blood pressure, headaches, racing heart, and so on. When you experience these side effects, simply back off on the amount of vitamin K you are taking, until the side effect disappear

8: About The Author And Other Resources

Rudy Silva is a natural consultant nutritionist educated in the United State of Nutrition and Physics. He is a graduate of San Jose State University in California. He is the author of 30 other e-books on natural remedies. He has authored a newsletter in natural remedies for over 4 years. He has many websites promoting special recommended products and information.

Resource page

To see all of the books written by this author, go to the internet and type Rudy Silva Articles in Google.

If you need support or want to promote any of his e-books, please contact him at rss41@yahoo.com and expect a reply within 24 hours. He looks forward to hearing from you and is happy to help you understand his material on natural and nutritional health.

Give a Review

And, don't forget to give a review for this book so that others can gain the benefits of what is in this book.

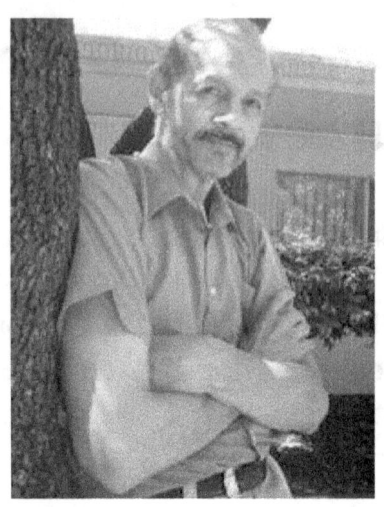

To you, for creating better health and more happiness in your life,

Rudy S Silva

Your doctor or health provider should confirm any information given here. This information should not be taken as medical advice or treatment. This e-book is for information and educational purposes only.